Birth Wizard's

Prenatal

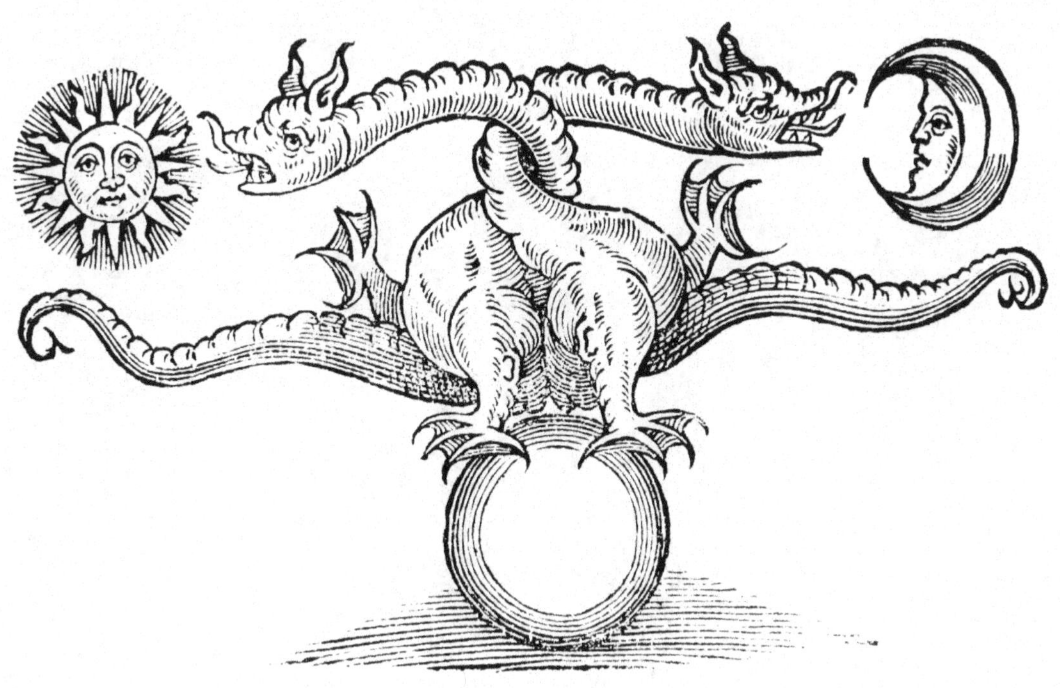

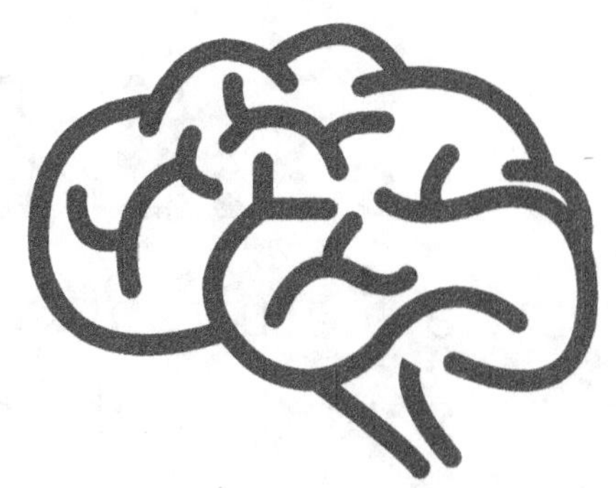

FIRST
THING
THAT
COMES
TO MIND

B/W

LET'S DRAW

Draw a picture of your birth. Put everything from smells, sounds, lighting, colors, feelings.. be abstract

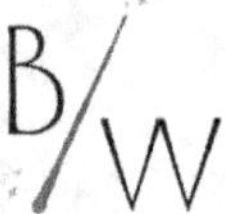

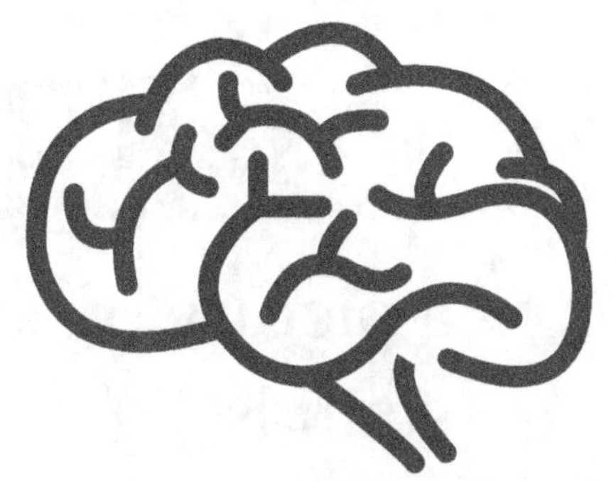

FIRST
THING
THAT
COMES
TO MIND

B/W

LET'S DRAW

Draw a picture of your birth. Put everything from smells, sounds, lighting, colors, feelings.. be abstract

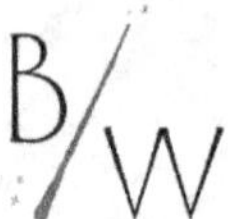

Body, Brain & Baby

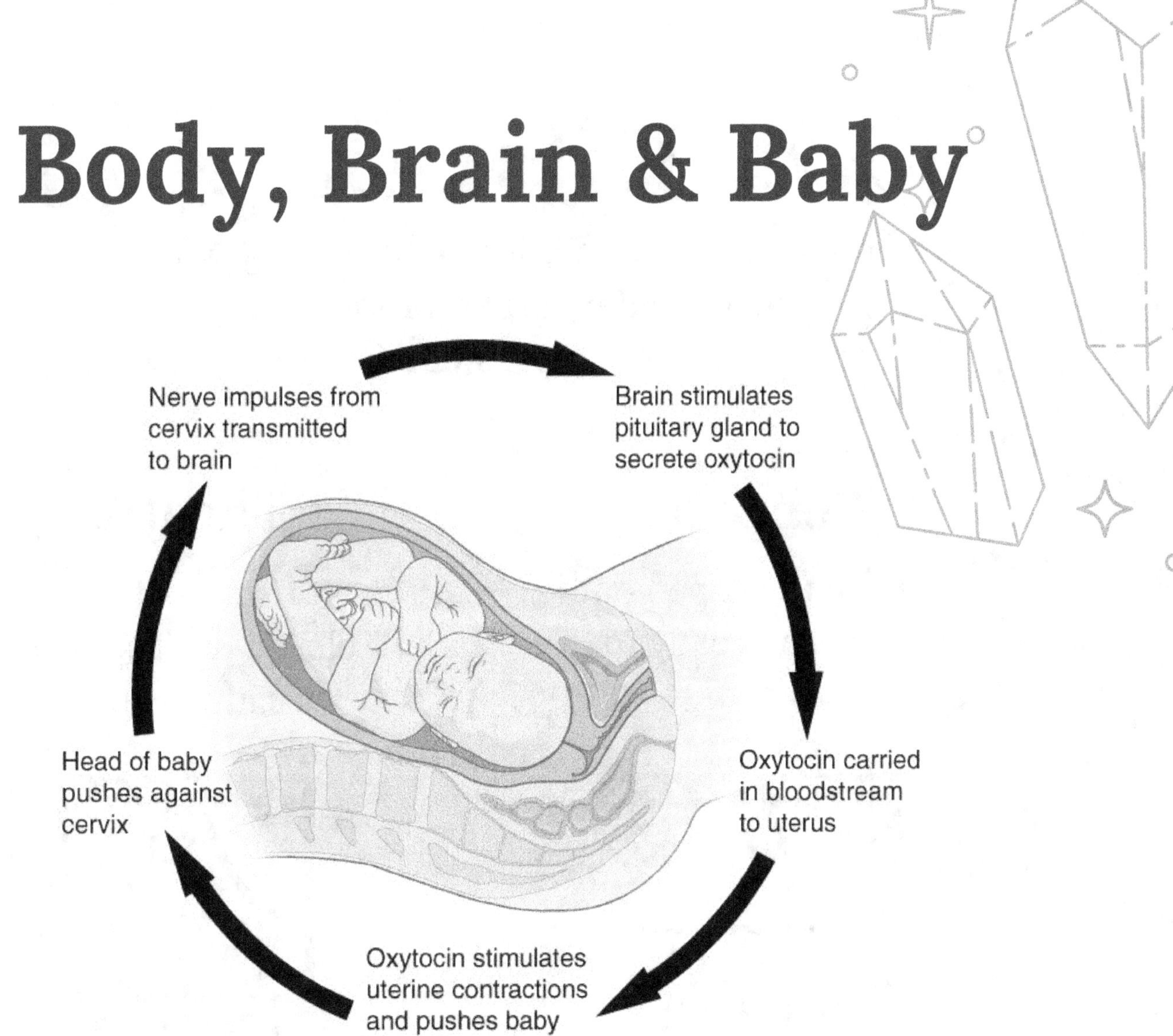

Something magical between the placenta, our blood stream & our brain.

~36 weeks, our brain tells our body to start being more sensitive to oxytocin.

~38 weeks, baby's will "drop" and nestle deeper against the cervix.

Positive feedback loop of labor relies on upright natural positions where the baby's head is encouraged to push against the cervix.

Dilation

the action or condition of becoming or being
made wider, larger, or more open.

0-10 cm

Concert

Curtains are open but
show isn't ready to
start

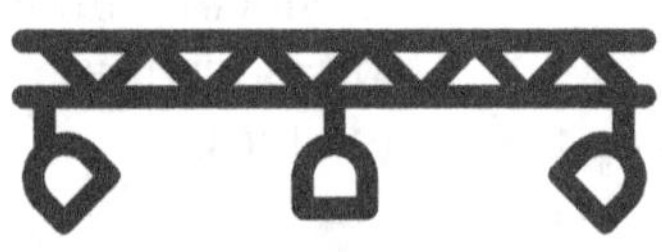

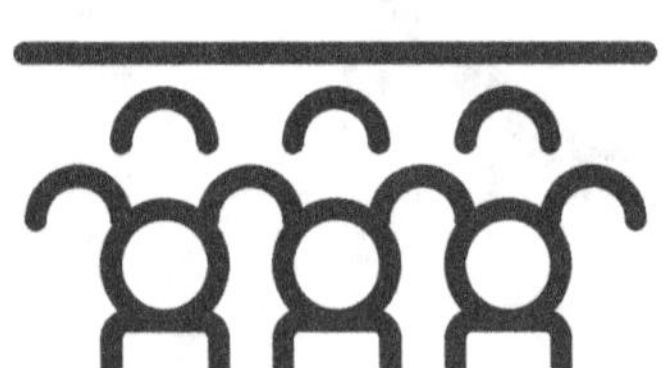

Theatre

Curtains stayed
closed until show is
ready to start

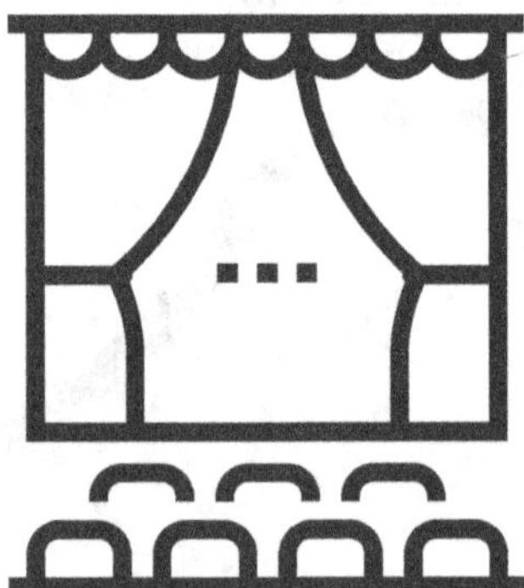

CERVICAL DILATION

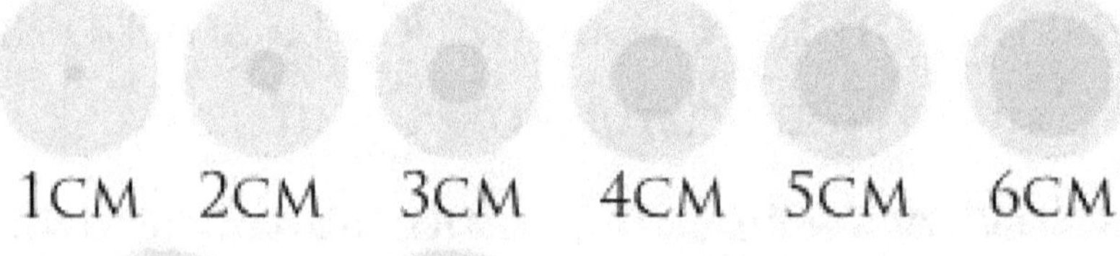

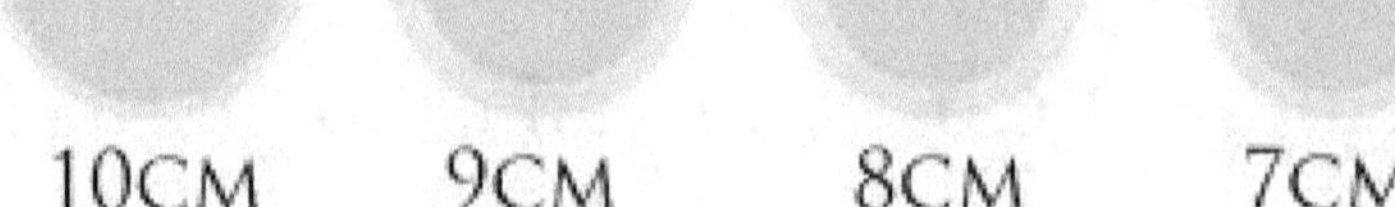

STATION

the baby's presenting part–most likely the head–
in relation to the ischial spines of the birther's
pelvis

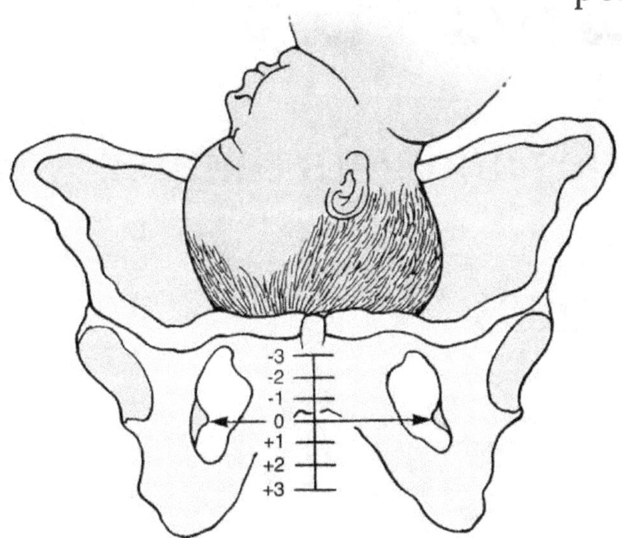

Understood on a number line
-3 to +3

Just like a train has stops at the
stations

Most major stop is 0

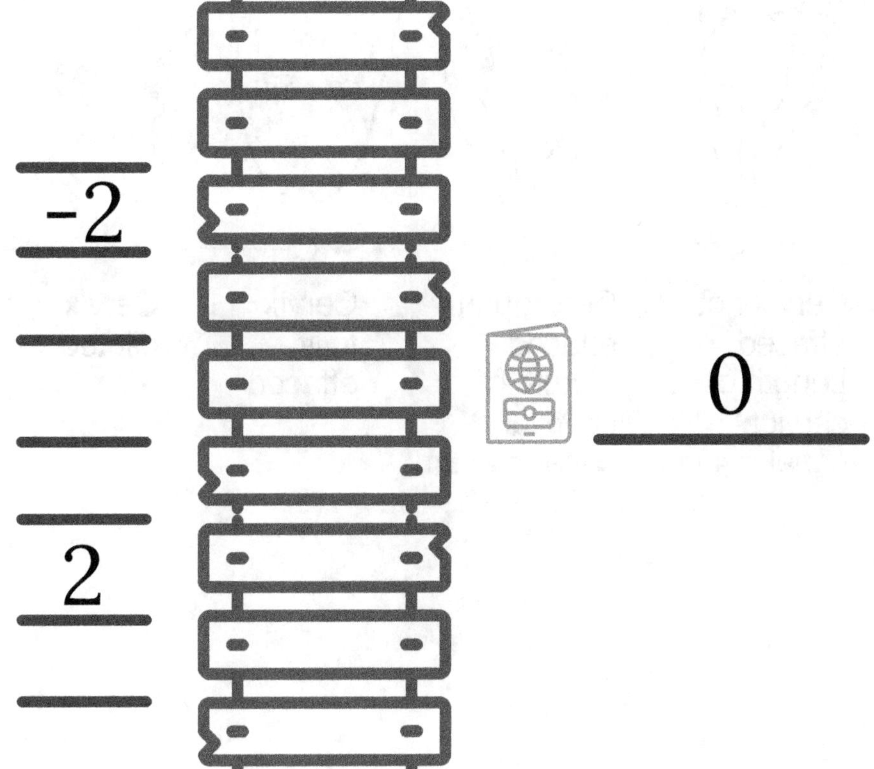

EFFACEMENT

that the cervix stretches and gets thinner

0% to 100%

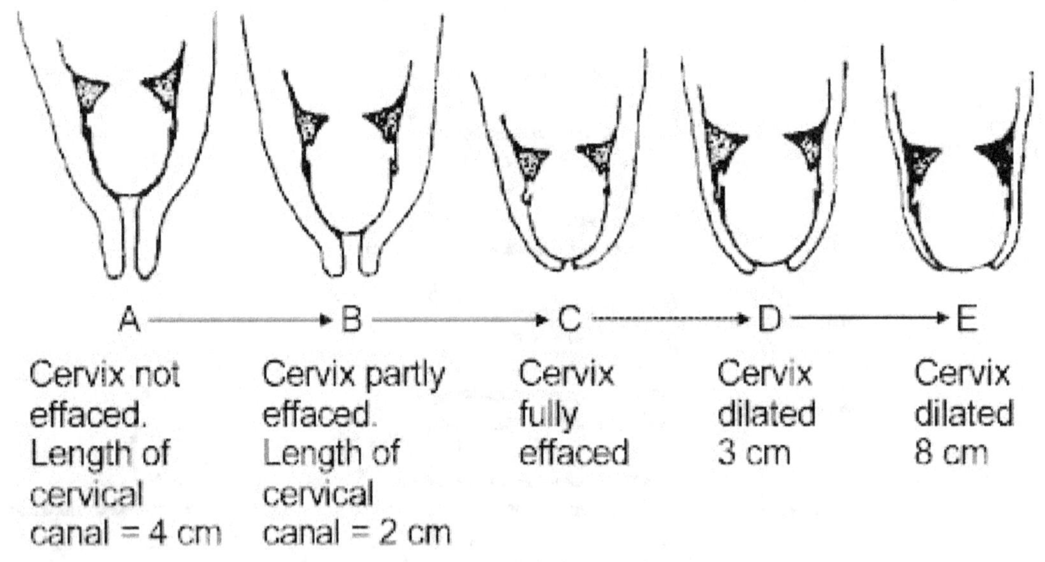

BOOK OF LABOR

Just like a book theres chapters to the stages
of labor

Some Chapters you will fall asleep through or
have a hard getting through them

Other Chapters you will wiz through them

No matter what you will finish the book

Preamble
Chapter 1- Early labor
Chapter 2-Bridging
Chapter 3-Active

Chapter 4- Transition
Chapter 5- Pushing
Chapter 6-Baby!
Chapter 7-Placenta

Preamble
Circle the ones you have experienced before

Loose-feeling joints

Bloody Show

Water Breaks

Baby Drops

Diarrhea

Instinct tells you its going to happen

Weight Gain Stops

Nesting

Losing Mucus Plug

Prodromal Labor

Fatigue

Lighting Crouch/Quickening

Chapter 1: Early Labor

Contractions may have regular pattern and easy to manage

Feelings	Contractions	Things to do
Excited	5-20 mins apart	Eat
Nervous	Not Consistent	Sleep
Annoyed	Can be ignored	Walk
		Go out
		Distraction

Dilation
0 cm to 4 cm

Effacement
0% to 60%

Chapter 2: Bridging

not clinically in "Active Labor" but you'll feel that way

Feelings

Like you are working
No longer "fun" but not bad
Annoyed
Excited
May Need support

Contractions

5-10 mins apart
Consistent
Managable

Dilation

2 cm to 5 cm

Effacement

20% to 60%

Things to do

Call doula or support

Leaning forward during
contractions may help

Still hanging out in intial
birth space

Chapter 3: Active

Progress is faster now, more intense

Feelings

Focused
Intensity
Rhythm
Intimidation
Confident

Contractions

2-4 mins apart
Consistent
Intensity picked up

Dilation

3 cm to 8 cm

Effacement

40% to 90%

Things to do

Call doula or support
Stairs
Hip circles
Moaning
Kissing
Dancing
Head to birthing space

Chapter 4: Transition
The last bit of dilation and can be overwhelming

Feelings
Fear
Encouragement
Accomplishment
"Finally"
Powerful/less

Contractions
2-3 mins apart
Consistent
Most Intense

Dilation
7 cm to 9 cm

Effacement
100%

Things to do
Routine
Tub or Shower
Zone Out
Breathe Deeply
Listening to baby/body

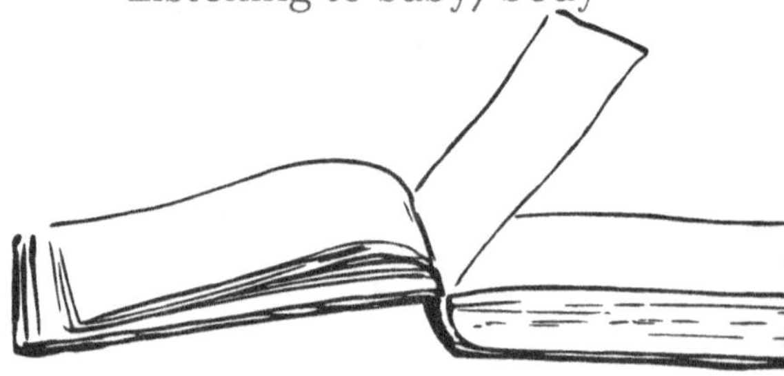

Chapter 5: Pushing
Complete and feeling pressure

Feelings
Surreal
Tired or Invigorated
Focus
Learning Curve

Contractions
2-3 mins apart
Consistent
Pressure

Dilation
10 cm

Effacement
100%

Station
+2 and beyond

Things to do
Changing Positions
Listening to body
Resting between
Breathing deep
Laboring down

On average a birther will push between 2-3 hours and change positions 6 times.

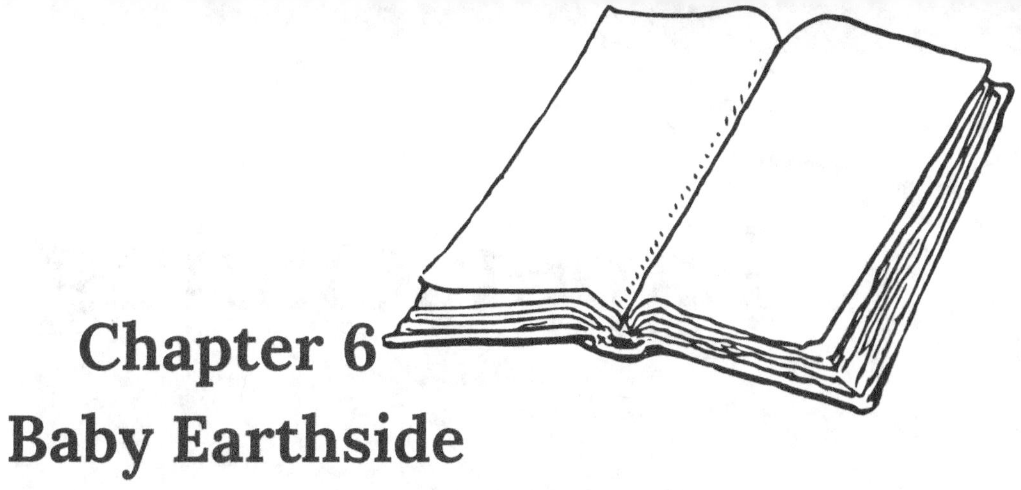

Chapter 6
Baby Earthside

You did
it!

Chapter 7: Placenta

Complete and feeling pressure

Feelings

Accomplished
Chills/Shakes
Oxytocin surge

Contractions

3-8 minutes
Similar to Early Labor

Things to do

Skin to Skin
Bodyfeed
Rest
Listening to body

Experiencing Labor

Pain Gate Theory

Activate your nerves in a non-painful way at the same time that you're experiencing pain, that that blocks the pain signals from reaching your brain.

Pain Vortex

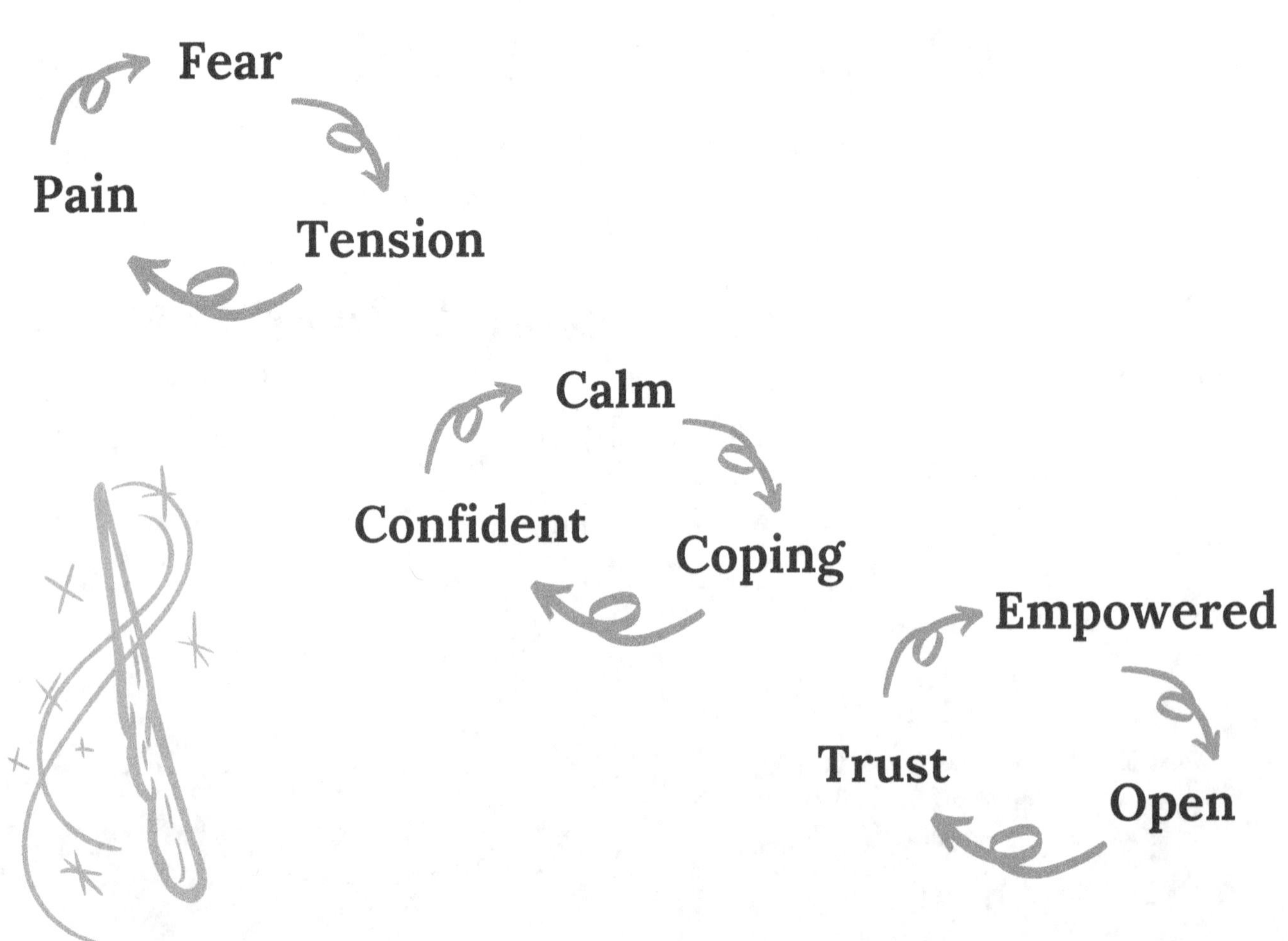

TOOLS FOR LABOR

Unmedicated
Circle ones you have or want to try

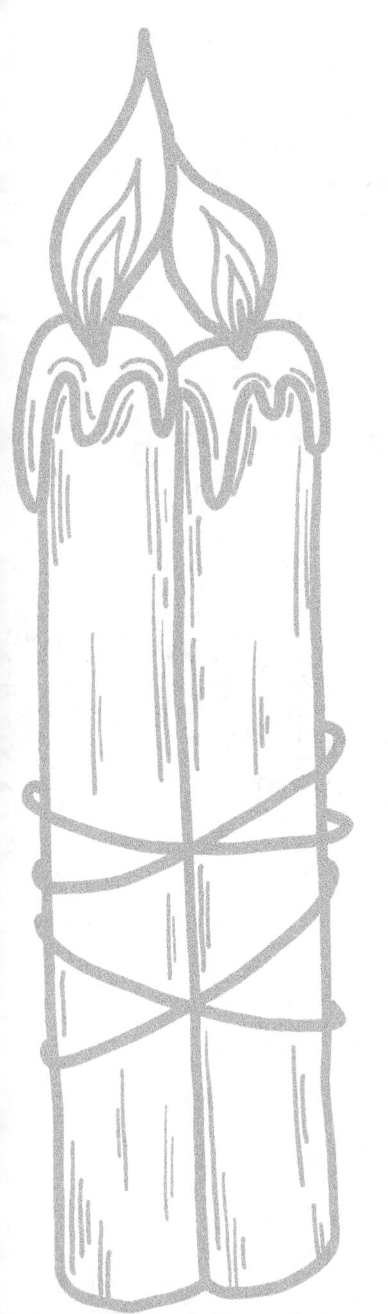

Comb

Birthing ball

Birth Stool

Walking

Dancing

Water

Jiggle

Aromatherapy

Breath

Growling

HypnoBirth/Babies

Acupuncture

Tens Unit

Double Hip Squeeze

Brushing Teeth

TOOLS FOR LABOR

Medicated

Epidural

an injection in your back to stop you
feeling pain in part of your body

Injected Opioids

used for acute, acute-on-chronic, or chronic
pain that cannot be controlled by other pain
management options

Nitrous Oxide

nitrous oxide is not a strong analgesic.
Birthers who use nitrous oxide during labor
may still have an awareness of labor pain.

Saline Shots

These injections are given into the person's lower back.
The onset of pain relief is fast, so it works pretty quickly
within about two minutes, and the pain management
effects can last as long as two hours

Therapeutic Rest

Therapeutic rest in labor involves administration of
parenteral analgesics in early or prodromal labor to
relieve the patient's discomfort

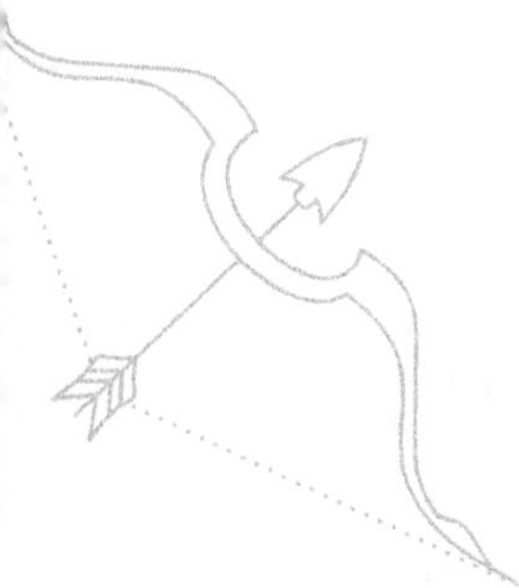

Party Members

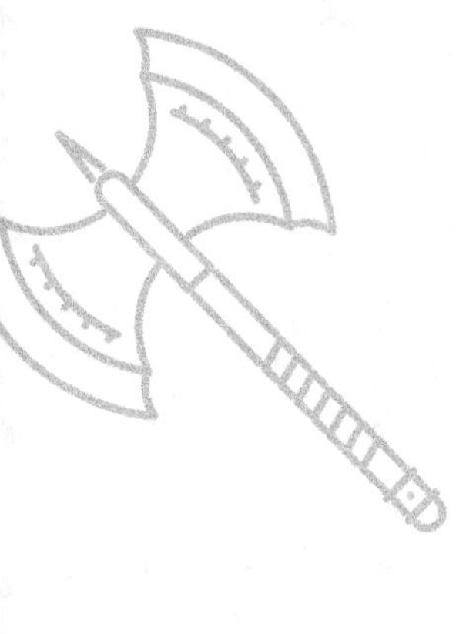

Name your qualities and skills only you
can bring to this quest

____

____

____

____

Name 3 birth wishes you hope to fulfill
during this quest

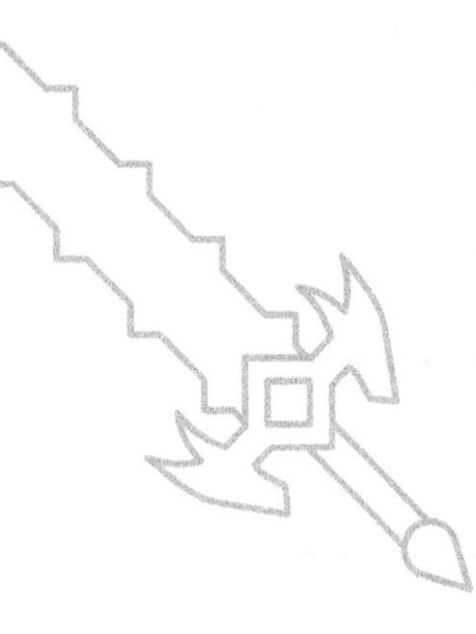

____

____

____

____

Advocating

Benefits

Risks

Alternatives

Intuition

Nothing

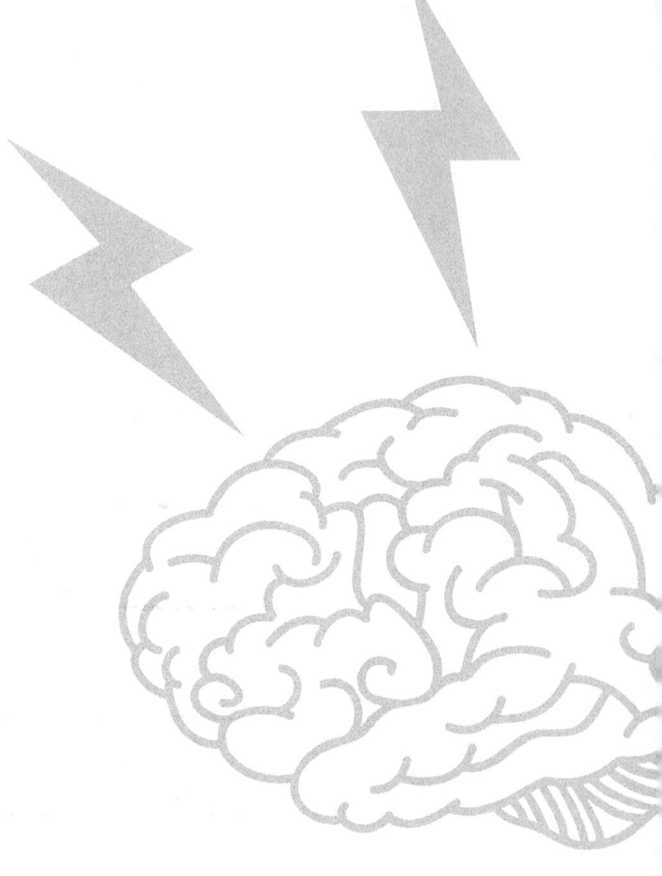

Safe Words

These can give you the oppertunity to slow down the room without signaling those making the space uncomfortable

What word do you want to use?

____

____

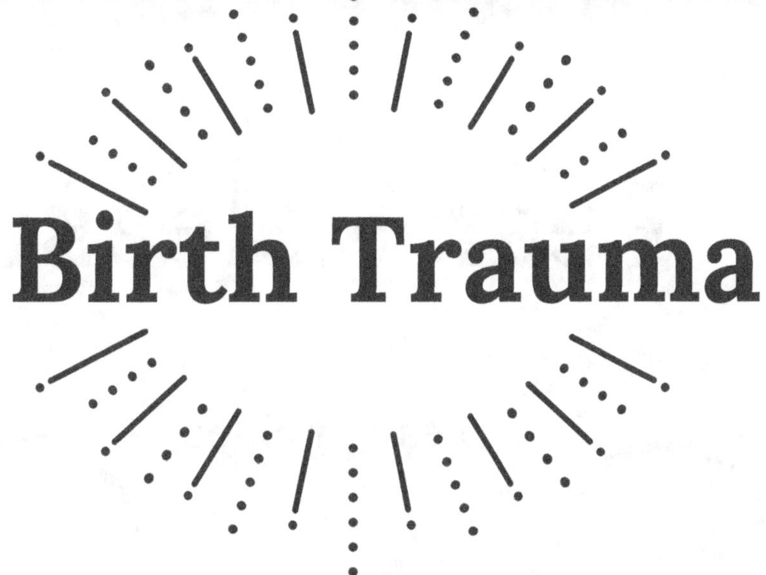

Birth Trauma

Stats say 7/10 birthing people will have a traumatic birth

Who is at risk?

Birthing complications

Birthing Interventions

Babies needing emergency care

People with significant injuries

People with pre-existing medical conditions

People with previous trauma and abuse

People from marginalized backgrounds

NO ONE IS IMMUNE!!

40% of people try a treatment approach and it doesn't work

Write 4 resources you can use in case of emergency

____

____

____

____

Fear Release

Fear Bubbles

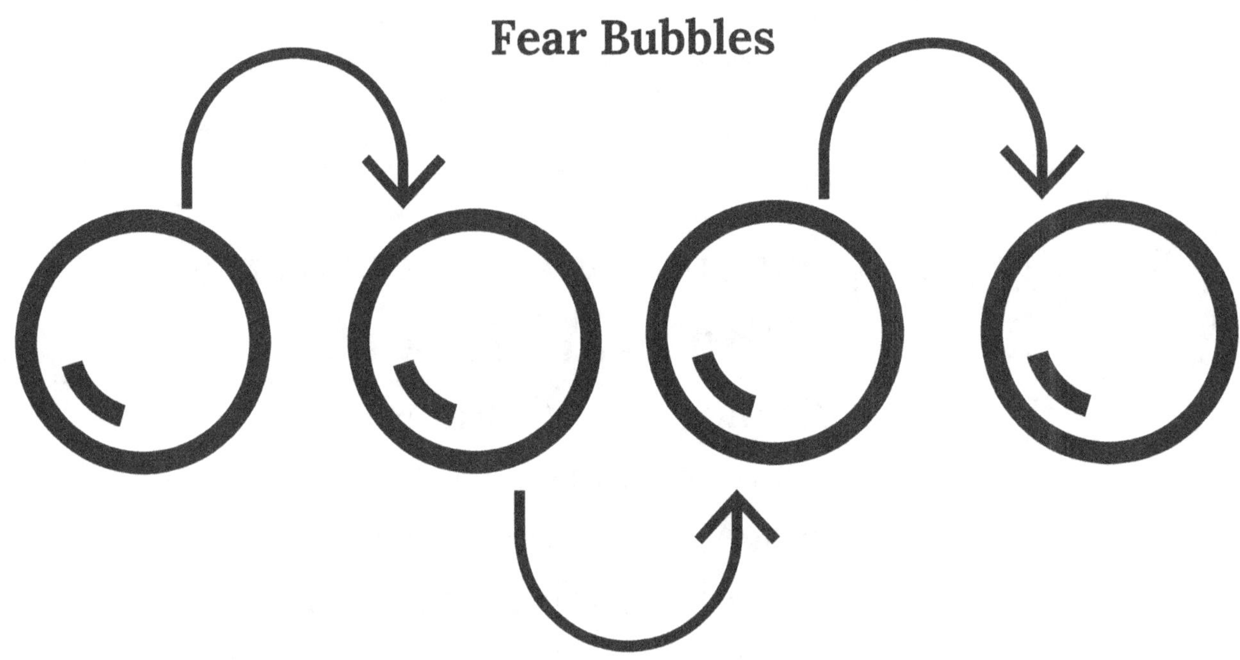

Breath Work

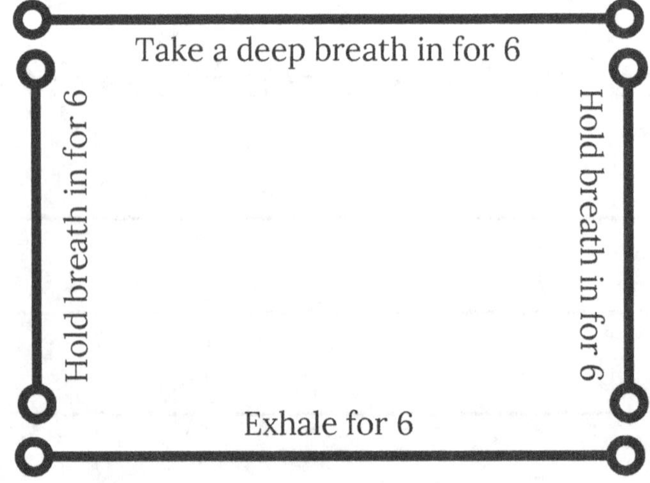

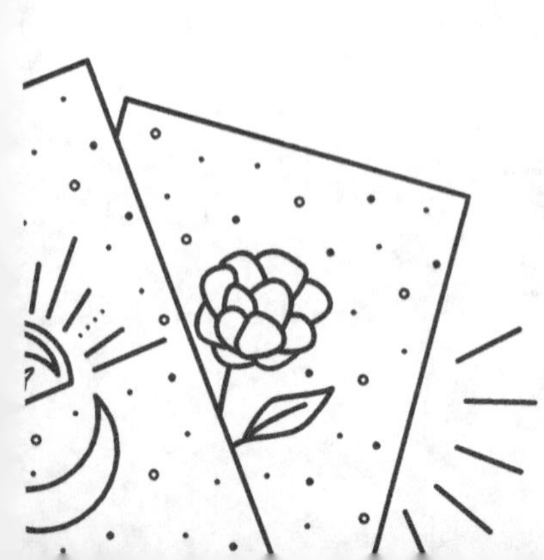

Cesarean Birth

Discuss with your VBAC Wizard

One Thing I need to know

One Thing I want to know

BABY

VAGINAL SEEDING
A swab to capture the flora to give to baby to help their gut

SKIN TO SKIN
Guaranteed to satisfy you!

DELAYED CORD CLAMPING
Allows for all the goodness from placenta to pass to baby by around 3 minutes after birth

BIRTHER

CLEAR DRAPE
A scrumptious classic, available at most hospitals but a good substitute is having baby peep over drape.

ESSENTIAL OILS & MUSIC
Double comfort measures for birther that can keep space more tranquil

NODES PLACED ON BACK
This allows for ease of movement and breastfeeding

PHOTOGRAPHY
Memories and honoring the moment with snapshots

SLIENCE
Not hearing the OR staff talk about their kid's soccer practice or upcoming vacation can keep the mood on point

SUPPORT

DOULA IN OR
The perfect sweetness to add to any OR

PARTNER STAYING WITH BABY
Our best-seller! This is an easy request that can fulfilled just about everytime.

BE SURE TO TALK PROVIDER ABOUT THEIR SECRET MENU

Birth Research

The purpose of Birth Planning is to allow you to research all your options. They allow you to understand backroads incase your journey hits a plot twist. Please take the time to use our light version of a birth plan for your own journey. It can be easily filled out and taken to your provider if you have further questions....

Birth Choices

Birth Name:

Partner:

Provider:

Pediatrician:

Baby Name:

Augmentation & Monitoring

- [ ] Movement
- [ ] Artificial rupture of membranes (AROM)
- [ ] Pitocin
- [ ] Cervidil/Cytotec
- [ ] Membrane Sweep
- [ ] a clear or lowered drape
- [ ] to have a slow delivery
- [ ] Intermittent Monitoring
- [ ] Continuous Monitoring
- [ ] Internal Monitoring

Pushing

- [ ] Perfer to wait to push until I feel the urge
- [ ] Mirror
- [ ] Coached Pushing
- [ ] Forceps
- [ ] Touch my baby's head as it crowns
- [ ] Pull baby out myself
- [ ] Have my partner catch baby
- [ ] Natural Tearing
- [ ] Use a variety of positions during pushing

Pain Management

- [ ] Movement
- [ ] Counter Pressue
- [ ] Water: Tub or Shower
- [ ] Nitrous Oxide
- [ ] Birth Ball
- [ ] Tens Unit
- [ ] Tramadol/Opioids
- [ ] Local Anesthesia
- [ ] Epidural

Baby & After Birth Care

- [ ] Delayed Cord Clamping
- [ ] Skin to Skin
- [ ] Vitamin K Shot/Drops
- [ ] Eye Ointment
- [ ] Breast/Chestfeeding   [ ] Formula
- [ ] Pitocin for bleeding
- [ ] Donate Placenta/Cord Blood
- [ ] Keeping Placenta
- [ ] Keep Baby in Room

Birth Choices

Birth Name:

Partner:

Provider:

Pediatrician:

Baby Name:

Prior to Birth, I would like

- ☐ to meet with members of the OR team who will be with me during delivery
- ☐ an explanation of the procedure before I am taken to the OR
- ☐ an explanation of the medications that will be used
- ☐ my partner/spouse/family member/doula to accompany me in the delivery room

For Pain Relief, I would like

- ☐ Epidural
- ☐ Spinal
- ☐ General Anesthesia

During Birth, I would like

- ☐ to wear my own labor and delivery gown
- ☐ to choose the music playing in OR
- ☐ ECG leads placed on my back
- ☐ my support to take pictures/video
- ☐ the procedure explained as it happens
- ☐ a clear or lowered drape
- ☐ to have a slow delivery
- ☐ Side Conversation limited
- ☐ No Students

Immediately following Birth, I would like

- ☐ my partner in the OR to announce the gender of our baby
- ☐ to delay cord clamping
- ☐ my spouse/partner to cut the umbilical cord
- ☐ immediate skin-to-skin on me or my partner
- ☐ vaginal seeding to be performed
- ☐ to have measurements/assessments performed while the baby is on my chest if they are needed immediately
- ☐ do not give me sedatives after the birth
- ☐ to see and touch the placenta and cord
- ☐ to have the opportunity to breastfeed in the OR

During Recovery, I would like

- ☐ a lactation consultant to visit
- ☐ my other children to come in to meet the new baby
- ☐ family to visit within 1-3 hours after birth
- ☐ my IV, catheter, ECG leads, etc. removed as soon as possible
- ☐ to eat and get up to use the restroom as soon as I feel ready and able to following delivery
- ☐ Limited interaction with nursing staff in night hours to allow rest and bonding
- ☐ a breast pump accessible in my room

Postpartum

S leep
N utition
O mega 3's
W alking
B aby breaks
A dult time
L iquids
L aughter

Resources that you'll need

____

____

____

Postpartum

	Hospital	Birth Center	Home
60 Minutes	Pitocin if needed Fundus Massage Skin to Skin Baby Tests	Pitocin if needed Fundus Massage Skin to Skin Meal Provided	Pitocin if needed Fundus Massage Skin to Skin Meal Provided
60 Hours	Typically Home Bleeding continues Milk shifting Hormone shifts/baby blues	Visit from Provider Bleeding continues Milk shifting Hormone shifts/baby blues	Visit from Provider Bleeding continues Milk shifting Hormone shifts/baby blues
60 Days	6 week postpartum appt 45-60 days ovulation occurs Cleared for usual activities	6 week postpartum appt 45-60 days ovulation occurs Cleared for usual activities	6 week postpartum appt 45-60 days ovulation occurs Cleared for usual activities

What are some of your plans for postpartum?

____

____

____

____

____

Postpartum

List ways your support
system can help you

____

____

____

____

____

____

____

____

____

Notes

Notes